Meal Prep

50 Simple Recipes For Health & Fitness Nuts

By

Marc McLean

Copyright 2017

By Marc McLean – All rights reserved

Author's Legal Disclaimer

This book is solely for informational and educational purposes and should not be considered a replacement for professional medical treatment. Please consult a medical or health professional in relation to all matters about your health.

The recipes in this book are not a prescription and do not make any claim about health improvements, or any difference to your health in its own right. There are many elements to good health, of which food is just one. The books does not offer medical advice and the author cannot be held responsibility for any injury or illness sustained while following the instructions in this book.

No part of this publication shall be reproduced, transmitted, or sold in any form without the prior written consent of the author.

Table of Contents

Introduction 1

Breakfasts 4

Main Meals 5

Souper Soups 6

Healthy Snacks 7

Power Shakes 8

Berry Crunch 9

Spiced-up Scrambled Eggs 10

Creamy Leeks & Eggs 11

Peanut & Banana Porridge 13

Hot Fruit & Nuts Cereal 14

Fruity Oats 15

Protein Pancakes 16

Broccoli Bake 17

Pepper & Onion Omelette 18

Quinoa Fruit Salad 19

Main Meals 20

    Turkey Chilli 21

Sweet Potato & Chickpea Curry 23

Paella Power 25

Creamy Garlic Pasta 27

Salmon & Veg Special 29

Chicken, Broccoli & Spinach Pie 31

Piri Piri Chicken 33

Veggie Chilli 35

Chicken Thighs With Sweet Potato 36

Chicken Satay Supreme 38

Soup-er Soups 41

Spiced Lentil & Vegetable Soup 42

Chicken & Rice Soup 44

Sweet Potato & Pepper Soup 45

Leek & Potato Soup 46

Pea, Leek & Bacon Soup 48

Creamy Carrot & Parsnip Soup 50

Salmon Soup 52

Creamy Chicken, Bacon & Potato Soup 54

Mixed Bean Soup 56

Split Pea & Courgette Soup 58

Healthy Snacks 60

    Nutty Protein Bars 61

    Coconut Protein Balls 63

    Simple Protein Cookies 64

    Sweet As A Nut Balls 66

    Choc Coconut Cookie Balls 67

    No Bake Brilliant Bars 68

    Cranberry & Coconut Balls 70

    Delicious Dates Bites 72

    Protein Raisin Cookies 73

    Almond Fudge Bars 75

Healthy Shakes 77

    Blueberry Blast 78

    Choc n' Banana 79

    Mango Monster 80

    Avocado Attack 81

    Strawberry Goji Smooth 82

    Tropical Twist 83

    Green Pineapple Power 84

    Ginger Booster 85

Chia Berry 86

Tropical Treat 87

About the author 88

Introduction

Cooking can be a pain in the @ss sometimes...

But so is the struggle to shift stubborn flab around your belly, or gain lean muscle, if you're not eating the right foods every day.

Your exercise efforts will go to waste if you don't back them up with good sources of protein, carbs and fats, and sufficient calories for your health and fitness goals.

No need to worry about that...because this book serves up 50 awesome recipes that are simple to make - and ridiculously tasty. These nutrient-packed recipes <u>make clean eating easy</u> and prove that you don't have to eat boring, bland food to get in great shape.

Each recipe also includes a calorie and macronutrients breakdown. Counting calories, carbs or grams or protein couldn't be easier.

Ready meals, takeaways, and most foods that come pre-packaged from the supermarket shelves don't do us any good. Processed to the point where they become 'dead foods' – i.e. most of the nutritional value has been stripped away, or they have been loaded with sugar, salt, additives and chemicals.

The answer – cook using fresh ingredients. Then you know exactly what is going into your meal and can take full charge of your daily nutrition.

I also want my meals to be as quick and easy as possible because...I'll be honest...I'm hardly a masterchef. But you don't have to be either to be able to prepare and produce tasty, healthy, fresh food.

I simply looked up lots of recipes, got loads more from friends, and just followed all the instructions and experimented a little along the way. I wasn't looking for Michelin star type meals, I just wanted recipes that ticked three boxes....

- Healthy
- Tasty
- Pretty easy to cook

After years of stuffing my face with some awesome grub, I've pulled together my best of the bunch. These include:

- 10 main meals (all ridiculously tasty)
- 10 breakfasts (with plenty of variety)
- 10 soup recipes (simple and delicious)
- 10 'power shake' recipes (jam-packed with vitamins and minerals)
- 10 healthy snacks (sooo good you wouldn't believe they're healthy)

Some recipes are very basic. Some are a *wee bit* more fancy...but you still won't find it difficult to cook them. Finally, the majority of recipes take less than 30 mins to prepare.

These are my personal favourite recipes...the ones I keep going back to. They're ideal for people who lift weights like me, or exercise regularly and are looking for nutritious food to not only fuel their workouts, but help their body repair, recover and develop afterwards.

I share these recipes with my online personal training clients who love most of them. (The sweet potato and chickpea curry main meal, and mango power shake, are among the favourites!) Freshly cooked meals will help keep your waistline trim, maintain good health, and help you sculpt a strong, athletic, awesome physique.

Enjoy!

Marc McLean

Online Personal Training & Nutrition Coach // Health & Fitness author // Food Lover

www.weighttrainingistheway.com

Meal Prep: 50 Simple Recipes For Health & Fitness Nuts

Breakfasts

Berry Crunch

Spiced-Up Scrambled Eggs

Creamy leeks and Eggs

Peanut Butter & Banana Porridge

Hot Fruit & Nuts Cereal

Fruity Oats

Protein Pancakes

Broccoli Bake

Pepper & Onion Omelette

Quinoa Fruit Salad

Main Meals

Turkey Chilli

Sweet Potato & Chickpea Curry

Paella Power

Creamy Garlic Pasta

Salmon & Veg Special

Chicken, Broccoli & Spinach Pie

Piri Piri Chicken

Veggie Chilli

Chicken Thighs With Sweet Potato

Chicken Satay Supreme

Souper Soups

Spiced Lentil & Veg

Chicken & Rice

Sweet Potato & Pepper

Leek & Potato

Pea, Leek & Bacon

Creamy Carrot & Parsnip

Salmon & Veg

Creamy Chicken, Potato & Bacon

Mixed Bean

Split Pea & Courgette

Healthy Snacks

Nut Protein Bars

Coconut Protein Balls

Simple Protein Cookies

Sweet As A Nut Balls

Choc Coconut Cookie Balls

No Bake Brilliant Bars

Cranberry Coconut Balls

Delicious Dates Bites

Protein Raisin Cookies

Almond Fudge Bars

Power Shakes

Blueberry Blast

Choc n' Banana

Mango Monster

Avocado Attack

Strawberry Goji Smooth

Tropical Twist

Green Pineapple Power

Ginger Booster

Chia Berry

Tropical Treat

Berry Crunch

Ingredients

1 cup natural Greek Yoghurt

1/4 cup blueberries

1/2 sliced banana

Handful of almonds

1/4 cup granola (aim for less than 20g of sugar per 100g)

Sprinkle of cinnamon

1 tsp of honey

Servings - 1

Nutrition per serving

Calories: 449

Protein: 31g

Carbs: 58g

Fat: 31g

Step 1

Pour the cup of natural Greek yoghurt into a bowl.

Step 2

Add the granola, banana slices, almonds, and blueberries.

Step 3

Sprinkle over the cinnamon and drizzle with honey.

Spiced-up Scrambled Eggs

Ingredients   **Servings - 1**

3 slices of thin chorizo slices/pepperoni slices

Nutrition per serving

3 eggs

2.5 tbsp butter   Calories: 712

2 slices wholemeal bread   Protein: 37g

1/2 white onion   Carbs: 36g

Roughly 1 tbsp grated cheddar cheese Fat: 44g

Sea salt and pepper

Step 1

Put 1.5 tbsp of butter in a saucepan over a low to medium low heat, dice the onion into small chunks and then cook it in the butter until soft.

Step 2

While the onion is cooking, cut the chorizo/pepperoni slices into small pieces and then add to the saucepan.

Step 3

Mix up the eggs in a bowl with 1/2 tsp of salt and just a small dash of pepper.

Step 4

Pour eggs into the saucepan, add grated cheese, and continue to cook on a low to low medium heat until ready.

Step 5

Serve with wholemeal toast.

Creamy Leeks & Eggs

Ingredients

4 leeks, chopped

3 tbsp butter

3 tbsp single cream

3 slices of crispy bacon

5 eggs

Servings - 2

Nutrition per serving

Calories: 364

Protein: 21g

Carbs: 28g

Fat: 18g

Step 1

Trim the leeks and then chopped into small square strips.

Step 2

Add 2 tbsp of butter to a saucepan and melt over a low heat.

Step 3

Add the leeks to the saucepan and cook for 5-6 mins until softened.

Step 4

Whisk 1 tbsp of single cream in a bowl together with the eggs, then season with salt and pepper.

Step 5

Melt the other tbsp of butter in another saucepan on a low heat, and then cook the eggs in it. Meanwhile, grill the bacon slices until they become crispy.

Step 6

Keep stirring the eggs so they don't become too firm. When the eggs are cooked, but still a little soft, divide them onto two plates.

Step 7

Add the other 2 tbsp of cream to the leeks and stir through.

Step 8

Top the eggs with the creamy leek mixture, then crumble the crispy bacon over the top.

Peanut & Banana Porridge

Ingredients

1/2 ripe banana

1 cup oats

1 cup almond milk or rice milk

1 tbsp natural unsweetened peanut butter

1 tsp honey

Servings - 1

Nutrition per serving

Calories: 507

Protein: 17g

Carbs: 79g

Fat: 16g

Step 1

Add the oats and almond milk to a saucepan and cook until the oats are softened and ready, adding more almond milk if necessary.

Step 2

Transfer the porridge oats to a large bowl and then slice up the half banana.

Step 3

Add the banana slices to the porridge, along with the tablespoon of peanut butter, and mix well.

Step 4

Drizzle a teaspoon of honey over the peanut and banana porridge mixture.

Hot Fruit & Nuts Cereal

Ingredients

1/2 cup almonds

1/2 cup cashews

1/2 ripe banana

1/2 tsp of ground cinnamon

Pinch of salt

100ml coconut milk

1 egg

Servings - 2

Nutrition per serving

Calories: 260

Protein: 9g

Carbs: 10g

Fat: 22g

Step 1

Add all ingredients to a blender or food processor and blitz until smooth.

Step 2

Warm the mixture on a medium heat for 5 mins.

Step

Serve and add almond milk, or some fresh berries, to suit your taste.

Fruity Oats

Ingredients

1 chopped pear

1/2 chopped apple

1 tbsp linseed

Handful of almonds

A splash of almond milk

1/2 cup oats

1 tsp honey

Servings - 1

Nutrition per serving

Calories: 454

Protein: 10g

Carbs: 73g

Fat: 11g

Step 1

Cook the oats as per instructions

Step 2

Meanwhile, chop the pear and apple into small chunks and place in a breakfast bowl, along with 6-8 almonds.

Step 3

Sprinkle the linseed over the fruit and pour over a little almond milk to moisten it.

Step 4

Pour the cooked oats over the fruit and nuts, then drizzle with honey and serve.

Protein Pancakes

Ingredients

3 medium free range eggs

1/2 cup oats

1 ripe banana

1 tbsp unsweetened peanut butter

1 tsp cinnamon

1-2 tsp honey

Servings - 3 pancakes

Nutrition per pancake

Calories: 229

Protein: 13g

Carbs: 36g

Fat: 12g

Step 1

Put the eggs, oats, cottage cheese, banana and cinnamon into a blender and mix into a batter consistency

(Add a bit more oats if it's too runny).

Step 2

Put a frying pan on at low to medium heat and pour the mixture in to cook pancakes.

Step 3

Drizzle the pancakes with honey and serve.

Broccoli Bake

Ingredients

8 broccoli florets

6 eggs

1 can / 400ml coconut milk

1 tbsp butter

1/2 cup grated cheddar cheese

1/4 tsp nutmeg

Salt and pepper

Servings - 4

Nutrition per serving

Calories: 347

Protein: 13g

Carbs: 5g

Fat: 31g

Step 1

Preheat the oven to 200°C/400°F/gas 6

Step 2

Cook the broccoli in boiling water for 5 mins until nearly softened.

Step 3

Butter a 10 inch round or small baking dish.

Step 4

In a large mixing bowl, whisk together the eggs, coconut milk, butter, nutmeg, salt and pepper.

Step 5

Drain the broccoli and stir into the mixing bowl, along with the grated cheese.

Step 6

Pour the mixture into the baking dish and cook for 20 minutes.

Pepper & Onion Omelette

Ingredients

3 eggs

1 red pepper, diced

1/2 white onion, diced

50g feta cheese, crumbled

1 tbsp extra virgin olive oil

Sea salt and pepper

Servings - 1

Nutrition per serving

Calories: 532

Protein: 31g

Carbs: 15g

Fat: 39g

Step 1

Add 1 tbsp of extra virgin olive oil to a frying pan at a low-medium heat.

Step 2

Add the diced pepper pan and cook for a few minutes, then add the onion and continue cooking until both are soft.

Step 3

Whisk the eggs in a bowl and season with salt and pepper to taste.

Step 4

Pour the eggs into the pan and cook on the low-medium heat for 2-3 mins.

Step 5

Crumble the feta cheese over the top of the eggs in the pan. Then put the pan under the grill until the eggs are cooked on top (be careful not to leave it under for too long and overcook them).

Quinoa Fruit Salad

Ingredients

1 cup quinoa

1 cup strawberries, sliced

1 cup blueberries, sliced

1 cup mango, diced

1 tbsp honey

1 lime

1 tbsp of chopped fresh basil

Servings - 4

Nutrition per serving

Calories: 272

Protein: 6g

Carbs: 60g

Fat: 3g

Step 1

Cook the quinoa as per instructions on the packet and then leave to cool for 10-15 mins.

Step 2

Mix the quinoa in a large bowl along with the sliced and diced fruit.

Step 3

Squeeze the juice of the lime into a small bowl and mix with the honey.

Step 4

Drizzle the lime and honey mixture over the quinoa and fruit. Garnish with the chopped basil.

Meal Prep: 50 Simple Recipes For Health & Fitness Nuts

Main Meals

- **Most meal recipes provide 4 servings.**
- **Why not make a batch at night and take another serving into work for lunch the next day?**
- **If there's the odd ingredient you don't like feel free to swap them to suit your tastes.**

Turkey Chilli

Ingredients

1 tbsp extra virgin olive oil

500g lean ground turkey

1 red onion, chopped

1 red pepper, chopped

1 green pepper

4 cloves garlic, minced

2 green chillies, diced

1 tsp of chilli powder

1 can red kidney beans

1 packet chilli seasoning mix

1 cup of water

Sea salt and pepper.

Servings - 4

Nutrition per serving

Quorn + rice

Calories: 376 489

Protein: 40g 28.5

Carbs: 24g 68

Fat: 13g 8.2

Step 1

Add the extra virgin olive oil to a large saucepan and heat at medium.

Step 2

Add lean ground turkey mince cook until brown on both sides.

Step 3

Add all the remaining ingredients and keep stirring regularly for 5-10 mins.

Step 4

Season with salt and pepper, then turn the heat up and bring the chilli to a boil.

Step 5

Cover the chilli with a lid, turn the heat down to low and simmer for 30 mins before serving.

Sweet Potato & Chickpea Curry

Ingredients

1 tbsp coconut oil

1 red onion, diced

1 red chilli, de-seeded and chopped

2 cloves garlic, minced

1 tsp ground ginger

1 tsp turmeric powder

1 tsp chilli flakes

1 tsp chilli powder

1/2 tsp cumin

1/2 tsp ground coriander

200g white rice

400g chopped tomatoes

400g chickpeas

400ml coconut milk

2 medium sweet potatoes, peeled and chopped

Sea salt and pepper

1 bunch fresh coriander

1 lime

230ml coconut yoghurt

Servings - 4

Nutrition per serving

Calories: 605

Protein: 14g

Carbs: 54g

Fat: 35g

Step 1

Cut the sweet potatoes into small chunks and cook in boiling water for 15 mins until softened.

Step 2

While the potatoes are cooking, heat the coconut oil in a large pan or wok, then add the onion and cook for a few minutes until softened. Add the garlic, chilli, ginger and spices, along with salt and pepper, then stir well and fry gently for a further couple of minutes.

Step 3

Add in the tomatoes, chickpeas and coconut milk. Stir and turn the curry down to a simmer. Finely chop a small handful of the coriander stems, then stir those in too, before adding the juice of half a lime.

Step 4

Cook the white rice or quinoa as per instructions on the packet.

Step 5

Add the sweet potatoes to the curry mix in the large pan. Cover with a lid for around 20 mins, stirring a couple of times and adding more seasoning and spices depending on your taste.

Step 6

Just before you're ready to serve, stir through the coconut yoghurt, along with more lime and spices if desired. Serve with the boiled rice or quinoa.

Paella Power

Ingredients

500g chicken breast

500g prawns

1tbsp extra virgin olive oil

3 cups short grain brown rice

400ml chicken stock

1/2 red onion

2 tomatoes

200g frozen peas

4 cloves garlic, minced

1 tablespoon of smoked paprika

Sea salt and pepper

Servings - 6

Nutrition per serving

Calories: 405

Protein: 42g

Carbs: 45g

Fat: 8g

Step 1

Cook rice according to the instructions on the packet and set aside.

Step 2

Chop chicken breasts into small chunks.

Step 3

Add the extra virgin olive oil to a wok or large skillet and warm up at a low-medium heat. Add the red onion and minced garlic, and cook until softened.

Step 4

Add in the chicken chunks, turn the cooker up to medium, and heat until the chicken is almost cooked through.

Step 5

Stir in the prawns and continue cooking for another 10 minutes.

Step 6

Add the paprika and sea salt and pepper to season. Stir well.

Step 7

Mix in the cooked rice, diced tomatoes, and keep stirring occasionally.

Step 8

Pour in the chicken stock and stir through.

Step 9

Add frozen peas in last and stir. Allow the paella to simmer for 5-10 minutes before serving.

Creamy Garlic Pasta

Ingredients

250g wholewheat penne pasta

400g cherry tomatoes, halved

2 medium shallots, sliced

8 garlic cloves, minced

2 tbsp extra virgin olive oil

4 tbsp of plain flour

400ml of almond milk

250ml of vegetable stock

Sea salt and pepper

Handful of fresh basil.

Servings - 3

Nutrition per serving

Normal Pasta

Calories: 280 — 494

Protein: 6g — 15.1

Carbs: 32g — 78.3

Fat: 12g — 13.2

Step 1

Preheat oven to 200°C/400°F/gas 6. Put the halved cherry tomatoes in a bowl and mix with the extra virgin

olive oil and sea salt.

Step 2

Place the tomatoes (cut side up) in a baking tray and cook in the oven for 20 mins.

Step 3

Add boiling water to a large saucepan and cook the penne pasta according to the instructions on the packet. Drain afterwards, cover and then set aside.

Step 4

In the meantime, add 1 tbsp of olive oil to a saucepan over a low-medium heat and then cook the garlic and shallots for a few minutes until softened. Season with salt and pepper.

Step 5

Stir in the flour and mix with a whisk. Slowly whisk in the almond milk a bit at a time so that clumps don't form. Then add in the vegetable stock.

Step 6

Add more salt and black pepper, turn up to a medium heat, and continue cooking for another 4-5 minutes to thicken.

Step 7

Keep stirring until the sauce reaches your desired thickness, then taste and add more salt and pepper if needed

Step 8

Add the pasta and roasted tomatoes and stir. Garnish with fresh basil.

Salmon & Veg Special

Ingredients

4 fresh skinless salmon fillets

2 large eggs

1 red onion, diced

2 garlic cloves, minced

3 tbsp extra virgin olive oil

2 tbsp red wine vinegar

200g asparagus, trimmed

100g garden peas

1 tsp finely chopped parsley

Sea salt and pepper

Servings - 4

Nutrition per serving

Calories: 437

Protein: 43g

Carbs: 3g

Fat: 26g

Step 1

Lightly grease kitchen foil on a baking tray and then place the salmon fillets on it.

Step 2

Season the salmon with salt and pepper before cooking in the oven at 180 degrees C / gas mark 4 for 12-15 mins.

Step 3

While the salmon is cooking, boil the eggs in a small saucepan. Then cool the eggs with cold water before cutting them into small, crumbly pieces.

Step 4

To make the vinaigrette, whisk together the diced red onion, red wine vinegar, olive oil and minced garlic in a mixing bowl. Season with salt and pepper.

Step 5

Bring a saucepan of salted water to the boil and cook the asparagus for 1 minute. Remove the asparagus, rinse with cold water and add to the vinaigrette, along with the garden peas.

Step 6

Sprinkle the chopped parsley into the vinaigrette bowl and toss the mixture.

Step 7

Place the salmon on plates, top with the vegetable mixture, and sprinkle the crumbled eggs over the top.

Chicken, Broccoli & Spinach Pie

Ingredients

2 skinless chicken breasts

6 broccoli florets

200g baby mushrooms, sliced

1/2 tsp of chilli flakes

Zest of 1 lemon

100g of spinach

8 sheets filo pastry

1 egg

25g butter

2 tbsp olive oil

Sea salt and pepper

Servings - 4

Nutrition per serving

Calories: 443

Protein: 26g

Carbs: 50g

Fat: 15g

Step 1

Preheat the oven to 180 degrees C / 350 degrees F. Place the chicken in a roasting tin, drizzled with 1 tbsp of olive oil and seasoned with salt and pepper. Cook for 20 mins until chicken is cooked through.

Step 2

While the chicken is in the oven, boil the broccoli in salted water for 10-15 mins until softened.

Step 3

Add 1 tbsp of extra virgin olive oil to a frying pan and cook the mushrooms on medium heat. Add the chilli flakes, lemon zest, and spinach and keep stirring until all the spinach is wilted.

Step 4

Stir the egg into the frying pan and season with salt and pepper.

Step 5

Cut the chicken into small chunks and add it to the spinach/mushroom mixture. Then mix in the broccoli.

Step 6

Brush a baking tin with butter and lay four sheets of filo pastry in the base to cover.

Step 7

Pour in half of the chicken and broccoli mixture, cover with two more filo pastry sheets, and then pour in the remaining chicken and broccoli mixture.

Step 8

Pull the sides of the pastry in, add the remaining sheets on top, and then tuck them down the sides of the pie.

Step 9

Brush the pastry with melted butter and mark the pastry into squares with a knife. Bake for 20 minutes 200°C/400°F/gas 6.

Piri Piri Chicken

Ingredients

4 chicken breasts

1 red pepper, sliced

1 yellow pepper, sliced

3 large sweet potatoes, diced

50g grated cheddar cheese

1-2 tsp ground oregano

6 sprigs of fresh thyme

1 red onion, diced

2 cloves garlic, minced

1 red chilli, diced

1 tbsp paprika

1 lemon

2 tbsp white wine vinegar

1 tbsp Worcestershire sauce

Sea salt and pepper

A bunch of fresh basil

Servings – 4

Nutrition per serving

Calories: 286

Protein: 26g

Carbs: 33g

Fat: 6g

Step 1

Slash the chicken breasts on each side a few times. Drizzle with olive oil, season with a little salt and pepper, and then cook in a griddle pan on a medium heat. Cook until golden underneath, then turn over.

Step 2

Peel and dice the sweet potatoes and boil in a saucepan of slightly salted water for 15 mins until softened.

Step 3

To make the piri piri sauce: add the red onion, garlic, chilli (stalks removed), paprika, the zest of 1 lemon and then its juice all together in a food processor. Add the white wine vinegar, Worcestershire sauce, bunch of basil, a couple of pinches of salt and pepper, along with a couple of splashes of water. Blend all ingredients until smooth.

Step 4

Add the sliced peppers to the pan alongside the chicken. Turn the heat down to low-medium and then turn the oven on to 200°C/400°F/gas 6.

Step 5

Pour the piri piri sauce into a casserole dish/roasting tray. Add the chicken and peppers to the tray next. Scatter over the sprigs of thyme, then put the tray into the middle of the oven.

Step 8

Drain the cooked potatoes and then mash them well in the saucepan, stir in the grated cheese, along with the oregano.

Step 9

Take the chicken out of the oven and check it's cooked through properly before serving alongside the potatoes.

Veggie Chilli

Ingredients

1 cup brown rice

400g pack of roasted vegetables

400g can of kidney beans, drained

400g can of chopped tomatoes

1 tsp medium chilli powder

1 tsp chilli flakes

1 green chilli, de-seeded and chopped

Sea salt and pepper

Servings - 2

Nutrition per serving

Calories: 472

Protein: 26g

Carbs: 80g

Fat: 10g

Step 1

Cook the rice in boiling water with some salt, according to instructions on packet.

Step 2

Preheat the oven to 200°C/400°F/gas 6. Cook the vegetables in baking tray for 15 mins until softened.

Step 3

Mixed in the kidney beans, chopped tomatoes, chilli powder, chilli flakes, and chopped green chilli. Stir through the vegetables and then season with some salt and pepper to suit your own tastes.

Step 4

Cook the veggie chilli mixture for another 10-15 mins in the oven.

Step 5

Drain rice and serve with the chilli.

Chicken Thighs With Sweet Potato

Ingredients

8 chicken thighs, skin on

1 tbsp mustard

1 tbsp honey

2 tbsp soy sauce

4 sweet potatoes, peeled and chopped

2 red peppers, chopped

1 tbsp extra virgin olive oil

Sea salt and pepper

100g baby spinach

Servings - 4

Nutrition per serving

Calories: 663

Protein: 42g

Carbs: 33g

Fat: 42g

Step 1

Preheat the oven to 200°C/400°F/gas 6. Boil the sweet potato slices in salted water for 5-6 mins until slightly softened then drain.

Step 2

Mix the mustard, honey and soy sauce together in a bowl, and season with salt and pepper.

Step 3

Mix the chicken thighs in the bowl until properly coated in the sauce.

Step 3

Heat the olive oil in a large frying pan over a medium heat. Cook the chicken, skin side down, in two batches for 4-5 mins until they start to brown. Turn over and cook the other side for 4-5 mins.

Step 4

Add the chicken to a roasting tin, along with the sweet potatoes and chopped peppers.

Step 5

Roast in the oven for 25 minutes until golden and the chicken is cooked through.

Step 6

Serve with washed baby spinach.

Chicken Satay Supreme

Ingredients

4 skinless chicken breasts

1 tsp of honey

1/2 small bunch of fresh coriander

1 fresh red chilli

1 clove of garlic, chopped

3 tbsp unsweetened peanut butter

2 tbsp soy sauce

1/2 tsp ground ginger

2 limes

(For the noodles)

250g thin egg noodles for pan frying

4 spring onions

2-3 cups bean sprouts

3 tbsp extra virgin olive oil

2 tbsp soy sauce

1 tsp brown sugar

Sea salt and pepper

Servings - 4

Nutrition per serving

Calories: 535

Protein: 54g

Carbs: 52g

Fat: 26g

Step 1

Turn the grill on to full and set out 4 metal skewers. (If you only have wooden ones soak them in water first).

Step 2

To make the satay sauce, put the following ingredients in a food processor: coriander, chilli (stalk removed), garlic, 3 tablespoons of peanut butter, 1/2 tsp of ginger, and a few splashes of soy sauce. Grate in the zest of both limes, then squeeze in the juice from 1 of them. Add a couple of splashes of water, a little salt and pepper, and then blend to a paste consistency.

Step 3

Spoon half of the satay sauce into a bowl, and the other half is to be used for the next step.

Step 4

Chop the 4 chicken breasts into small-medium sized chunks and then spear them with the skewers. Put them in a roasting tray and then use your hands to coat them well with half of the satay sauce.

Step 5

Drizzle the chicken with olive oil and season with sea salt. Put under the grill, for around 10 minutes on each side, or until golden and cooked through.

Step 6

While the chicken is cooking, rinse the spring onions and bean sprouts, and then chop the the spring onions into small pieces. Put the noodles in a large bowl, cover with boiling water and a plate, then leave to soak for 2-3 minutes.

Step 7

Mix the soy sauces, sesame oil, sugar, salt and pepper in a small bowl and set aside. Put a wok over a medium-high heat with a tablespoon of oil to coat it.

Step 8

Spread the noodles evenly in the wok and tilt it in a circular motion to spread the oil.

Step 9

Turn the chicken skewers over to cook the other side then return to the wok and turn the noodles over too once they become crisp. Flip them over and add another tablespoon of oil around the wok to cook the other side.

Step 10

Add the chopped spring onions, beansprouts and sauce to the wok and toss continuously. Cook for no more than 1 minute so that the sprouts remain crunchy.

Step 12

Plate up the chicken and noodles and serve.

Meal Prep: 50 Simple Recipes For Health & Fitness Nuts

Soup-er Soups

- **Easy to make soups with plenty of vegetables.**
- **Ready in under an hour and the most of the recipes provide 4 generous servings.**
- **Don't forget to season with salt and pepper to suit your own tastes.**

Spiced Lentil & Vegetable Soup

Ingredients

1 tbsp of extra virgin olive oil

1 tbsp of mild or medium curry powder

3 cloves of garlic, minced

2 litres of water

2 vegetable stock cubes

1 white onion, chopped

3 medium carrots, peeled and chopped

100g red lentils

1 parnsip, peeled and chopped

1 medium stalk of celery, chopped

1 tbsp of tomato puree

Sea salt and pepper

Servings - 4

Nutrition per serving

Calories: 115

Protein: 4g

Carbs: 20g

Fat: 3g

Step 1

Heat the oil in a soup pot, add the curry powder and garlic and stir over a low heat for 1 minute.

Step 2

Add the water, two stock cubes, the rest of the ingredients and bring to the boil.

Step 3

Turn the heat down and season with salt and pepper. Put the lid on and cook for 35-40 mins.

Step 4

Puree with a hand blender, or using a food processor, and then serve.

Chicken & Rice Soup

Ingredients

2 chicken legs with skin on

2 medium carrots, peeled and grated

1 white onion, chopped

1/2 cup white rice

2 chicken stock cubes

2 litres of boiling water

Sea salt and pepper

Servings - 6

Nutrition per serving

Calories: 213

Protein: 9g

Carbs: 14g

Fat: 7g

Step 1

Pour the boiling water into the soup pot and dissolve the stock cubes.

Step 2

Add the chicken legs, then the rice and bring to the boil.

Step 3

Add in the grated carrots and chopped onion, and turn the heat down, allowing the pot to simmer for 30-40mins.

Step 4

Remove the chicken legs carefully and cut off all the remaining chicken from the bone. Then chuck this back into the pot.

Step 5

Season the soup with salt and pepper to suit your own tastes, then serve.

Sweet Potato & Pepper Soup

Ingredients

1 tsp of coconut oil

2 large sweet potatoes, peeled and chopped

2 red onions, chopped

1 red pepper, chopped

4 cloves of garlic, minced

2 litres of vegetable stock

Sea salt and pepper

Chopped parsley

Servings - 4

Nutrition per serving

Calories: 100

Protein: 2g

Carbs: 21g

Fat: 2g

Step 1

Heat the oil in a large pot and fry the onion and garlic for 3 minutes on low heat. Add in the sweet potato, carrot and bell pepper and cook for 5 minutes on high. Stir occasionally.

Step 2

Add the water and the vegetable stock cubes, bring to boil and simmer the soup for 20 minutes.

Step 3

Puree the soup with a hand blender, and season with salt and pepper.

Step 4

Garnish with a little chopped parsley and serve.

Leek & Potato Soup

Ingredients

2 tbsp butter

3 leeks, sliced

1 white onion, chopped

250g potatoes peeled and diced

850 ml of vegetable stock

150ml of single cream

Salt and pepper

Servings - 4

Nutrition per serving

Calories: 251

Protein: 4g

Carbs: 27g

Fat: 14g

Step 1

Prepare are the vegetables, slicing the leeks, chopping the onion, and then dicing the potatoes.

Step 2

Add the butter to a large saucepan and melt it over a low heat.

Step 3

Add the vegetables to the saucepan and saute for 3-4 mins until soft but not brown.

Step 4

Pour in the vegetable stock, increase the heat on the cooker and bring to the boil.

Reduce the heat, season with salt and pepper, and then simmer for 15 mins.

Step 5

Turn off the cooker and liquidise with a hand blender. Alternatively pour into a blender machine and blitz until smooth.

Step 6

Mix in the single cream and then serve.

Pea, Leek & Bacon Soup

Ingredients   **Servings - 4**

2 litres chicken stock (use 2 stock cubes)

Nutrition per serving

2 medium potatoes, peeled and chopped

2 leeks, chopped   Calories: 289

450g frozen garden peas   Protein: 12g

8 slices of smoked bacon, grilled to crispy   Carbs: 42g

chopped into strips

Fat: 8g

Step 1

Cook the 8 slices of bacon under the grill until crispy and set aside.

Step 2

Add the chicken stock cubes to a soup pot and dissolve them with the boiling water.

Step 3

Add in the potatoes and cook for 5 minutes. Next add the sliced leek and let everything boil for 10 minutes.

Step 4

Add in the peas and cook for another 5 mins. Season with salt and pepper then puree everything with a hand blender.

Step 5

Cut the bacon into small strips, mixing the majority of it through and garnishing with a few pieces.

Creamy Carrot & Parsnip Soup

Ingredients

2 tbsp butter

500g carrots, peeled and chopped

2 large parsnips, peeled and chopped

1 large onion, chopped

800ml of vegetable stock

150ml single cream

2 tsp of ground ginger

Grated zest of 1 orange

Salt and pepper

Fresh coriander, to garnish

Servings - 4

Nutrition per serving

Calories: 262

Protein: 4g

Carbs: 30g

Fat: 15g

Step 1

Put a large saucepan on a low heat and melt the butter.

Step 2

Add the chopped onion and cook for 3-4 mins until softened, then add the chopped carrots and parsnips.

Cover the saucepan and cook for 15 minutes, stirring occasionally.

Step 3

Add the ginger, orange zest and stock, then season with salt and pepper.

Step 4

Bring to the boil, then reduce the heat and simmer for 30 minutes until the vegetables are soft.

Step 5

Turn the cooker off and allow the soup to cool for 15 minutes. Then, either using a hand blender or

transferring to a food processor, blitz the soup until smooth.

Step 6

Mix in the cream and, when serving, garnish with fresh coriander.

Salmon Soup

Ingredients

2 tbsp butter

1 leek, sliced

1 large onion, chopped

850ml fish stock

1 large potato, peeled and chopped

1 tbsp plain flour

300g salmon fillets (skin removed), chopped into small chunks

2 egg yolks

1 tbsp chopped parsley

1 tbsp chopped dill

100ml single cream

Servings - 4

Nutrition per serving:

Calories: 311

Protein: 22g

Carbs: 23g

Fat: 15g

Step 1

Prepare all the vegetables and leave to one side. Add the butter to a large pan and melt over a medium heat.

Step 2

Add the leek and onion and then cook for 3-4 mins on a medium heat until softened.

Step 3

Mix the flour with a little vegetable stock until it makes a paste and then stir into the saucepan.

Step 4

Cook for a couple of minutes and then add in the rest of the vegetable stock, along with the parsley and dill, while stirring throughout.

Step 5

Season with salt and pepper, turn up the heat and then bring to the boil.

Step 6

Reduce the heat and let the soup simmer for 20 mins.

Step 7

Add the salmon chunks and cook for 6-8 mins until cooked through.

Step 8

Whisk together the egg yolks and cream in a bowl, and then stir into the soup. Cook for another 10 mins and then serve.

Creamy Chicken, Bacon & Potato Soup

Ingredients

1 tbsp butter

1 large onion, chopped

3 leeks, sliced and chopped

250g smoked lean bacon, chopped

700g potatoes

2 tbsp plain flour

1 litre chicken stock

3 garlic cloves, chopped

200g skinless chicken breast, diced

4 tbsp double cream

Sea salt and pepper

Fresh parsley

Servings - 4

Nutrition per serving

Calories: 520

Protein: 40g

Carbs: 46g

Fat: 17g

Step 1

Add the butter to a large saucepan and melt over a low heat.

Step 2

Add the onion, leeks and garlic, and cook for 3-4 minutes until softened. Then add in the bacon and allow it to cook through.

Step 3

In a bowl, mix the flour with some of the vegetable stock, enough to make a paste. Stir the paste into the saucepan and then cook for 2-3 minutes, while stirring.

Step 4

Pour in the the remaining stock, and add in the potatoes and diced chicken. Season with salt and pepper afterwards.

Step 5

Bring to the boil, then lower the heat and simmer for 25-30 mins until the chicken and potatoes are well cooked.

Step 6

Stir in the double cream and leave to cook for a few more minutes. Meanwhile, grill a slice of bacon until crispy.

Step 7

Serve the soup and garnish with the crispy bacon and parsley.

Mixed Bean Soup

Ingredients

1 tbsp extra virgin olive oil

4 spring onions, chopped

3 garlic cloves, chopped

200g mushrooms, sliced

1 large carrot, peeled and chopped

400g canned mixed beans, drained

800g (2 cans) chopped tomatoes

1 litre vegetable stock

1 tbsp thyme

1 tbsp oregano

4 tbsp double cream

Salt and pepper

Servings - 4

Nutrition per serving

Calories: 262

Protein: 9g

Carbs: 29g

Fat: 13g

Step 1

Add the extra virgin olive oil to a large saucepan and heat at medium.

Step 2

Add the prepared garlic and spring onions, and cook for 3-4 mins until softened.

Step 3

Add the mushrooms, carrots, chopped tomatoes, mixed beans, and vegetable stock.

Step 4

Season with salt and pepper and then bring to the boil.

Step 5

Lower the heat and then simmer for 30 minutes. Then turn off the heat and allow the soup to cool for 15 mins.

Step 6

Either using a hand blender, or by transferring the soup into a food processor, blitz the soup until smooth.

Step 7

Stir in the cream, heat for two more minutes, and then serve.

Split Pea & Courgette Soup

Ingredients

1 large white onion, chopped

2 medium courgettes, diced

200g yellow split peas

1 tbsp extra virgin olive oil

850ml vegetable stock

1/2 tsp turmeric

Sea salt and pepper

Servings - 4

Nutrition per serving

Calories: 153

Protein: 7g

Carbs: 19g

Fat: 5g

Step 1

Put the split peas in a bowl and a pint of water. Allow to soak for a 3-4 hours. Drain the split peas and rinse them before draining again.

Step 2

Add the extra virgin olive oil and heat in a large saucepan at medium.

Step 3

Add in the courgettes and onion, and cook for 3-4 minutes until softened.

Step 4

Pour in the vegetable stock, add the split peas and turmeric, and then bring to the boil.

Step 5

Reduce the heat, season with salt and pepper, and then simmer for 35-40 mins until the split peas are properly cooked through.

Healthy Snacks

- **10 tasty snacks all ridiculously easy to make.**
- **Where protein powder is included in recipes, I recommend <u>plant-based</u> protein (i.e. Sunwarrior or Vegan Blend from MyProtein.com) rather than whey protein powder.**

Nutty Protein Bars

Ingredients

Servings - 5

2 scoops of chocolate protein powder

Nutrition per serving

2 tbsp of oats

2 tbsp of linseed   Calories: 275

2 handfuls of crushed walnuts   Protein: 22g

2 tablespoons of organic unsweetened peanut butter

Carbs: 13g

4oz (half a glass) of almond milk   Fat: 13g

1 tbsp of Stevia

1 tsp of cinnamon powder

Step 1

Add the protein powder, oats, linseed, seeds, Stevia and cinnamon powder to a bowl. Then mix it all up with a spoon. Like a boss.

Step 2

Add the almond milk to moisten the mixture. You may need to add a little more almond milk, but you don't want it to be too runny. Next add in the two tablespoons of peanut butter and stir it thoroughly into the mixture.

Step 3

The peanut butter will help congeal the mixture. Now use your hands to push it all together firmly and roll it into a big ball.

Step 4

Rip chunks of the mixture off the ball and shape them into bars. (You should be able to make 4 decent sized ones with this amount of ingredients).

Step 5

Place them on a foil baking tray and use a little olive oil or butter to grease the bottom so the protein bars don't stick when cooked. Bake at 200°C/400°F/gas 6 for 25-30 mins.

Step 6

Whip your amazing cooking creations out of the oven and smell those little beauties. Forget the fact that they look like baked turds….because they taste awesome.

Coconut Protein Balls

Ingredients

1 cup cashew nuts

1 cup of dates

1 scoop of chocolate protein powder

1 tbsp desiccated coconut

Servings - 6

Nutrition per serving

Calories: 224

Protein: 8g

Carbs: 27g

Fat: 10g

Step 1

For 10 minutes soak the dates in boiling water.

Step 2

Blend the cashew nuts in a food processor.

Step 3

Drain the dates and add them to the food processor with the cashews. Blend until they start to clump together.

Step 4

Next add in the protein powder and blitz until it starts to get crumbly and then clump together again.

Step 5

Roll the mixture into 4 balls with your hands.

Step 6

Scatter the desiccated coconut on parchment paper and roll the balls in it. Place them in a plastic tub and store in the fridge.

Simple Protein Cookies

Ingredients

1 cup oats

2 scoops of chocolate protein powder

1/3 cup unsalted peanuts

1/4 cup coconut oil, melted

2 tbsp unsweetened peanut butter

4 dates, pitted

Cup of water

Servings - 8

Nutrition per serving

Calories: 207

Protein: 9g

Carbs: 12g

Fat: 14g

Step 1

Mix together the oats, peanuts and protein powder in a large mixing bowl.

Step 2

Add the peanut butter, coconut oil, dates and water to a blender and blitz until smooth.

Step 3

Pour this blender mixture into the bowl with the dry ingredients and mix well together. This should be quite thick but add a little more water if there are some dry patches in the bowl.

Step 4

Scoop this cookie mix out onto a chopping board and roll into balls slightly bigger than golf balls, then flatten with your hands.

Step 5

Place the cookies on a baking sheet and put in the fridge for 1 hour to harden before eating.

Sweet As A Nut Balls

Ingredients

1 cup unsweetened almond butter

1/3 cup of coconut cream concentrate melted

3/4 cup of raisins

1/2 cup sunflower seeds

Servings - 8

Nutrition per serving

Calories: 188

Protein: 4g

Carbs: 16g

: 12g

Step 1

Put all ingredients in a food processor and blitz until smooth.

Step 2

Roll into individual balls and place on parchment paper.

Step 3

Place the balls in a plastic tub and refrigerate for 30-60 mins until they harden and are ready to eat.

Choc Coconut Cookie Balls

Ingredients	**Servings - 10**
1/2 cup coconut flour	**Nutrition per serving**
2 scoops chocolate protein powder	
2 tsp baking powder	Calories: 99
4 packets Stevia extract	Protein: 7g
2 tbsp desiccated coconut	Carbs: 6g
1/4 tsp sea salt	Fat: 5g
1/2 tsp cinnamon	
2 egg white	
1 tbsp vanilla extract	
1/4 cup almond butter	
1/4 cup almond milk	
1/4 cup mini dark chocolate chips	

Step 1
Preheat oven to 180°C/350°F/gas 4. First mix all the dry ingredients in a bowl and then blend in the wet ingredients, mixing with a wooden spoon.

Step 2
Roll into 12 small round balls and place on a baking sheet lined with parchment paper.

Step 3
Bake for 8-10 minutes or until golden brown.

Step 4
Leave to cool for 10 minutes and then serve.

No Bake Brilliant Bars

Ingredients

3 cups of brown rice cereal

2 tbsp honey

2 tbsp unsweetened peanut butter

2 scoops of chocolate protein powder

1/2 cup cashews, crushed

2 tbsp chocolate chips

Servings - 10

Nutrition per serving

Calories: 180

Protein: 8g

Carbs: 22g

Fats: 5g

Step 1

Line a baking tray with parchment paper.

Step 2

Heat a small saucepan on a low heat and add the honey and peanut butter, stirring regularly. Cook for a few minutes until they are melted and well mixed together.

Step 3

Add in the brown rice cereal, protein powder, crushed cashews, and stir everything together for 2-3 minutes. Turn the cooker off and then add in the chocolate chips last (so they don't melt).

Step 4

Using a wooden spoon, transfer the mixture onto the lined baking tray. Place another piece of parchment paper on top and the press down with your hands until the mixture is even as possible.

Step 5

Put in the fridge for 4-5 hours, or overnight, then remove the parchment paper and cut into 10 bars.

Cranberry & Coconut Balls

Ingredients

1/2 cup cranberries

5 medjool dates, pitted

1/2 cup fruit and nut mix

1/2 cup almond flour

1/3 cup coconut flour

2 tbsp chia seeds

2 tbsp coconut oil, melted

2 tbsp honey

2 scoops chocolate or vanilla protein powder

2 tbsp desiccated coconut

Servings - 12

Nutrition per serving

Calories: 168

Protein: 8g

Carbs: 21g

Fat: 7g

Step 1

Add the cranberries, dates, and fruit and nut mix to a food processor and blitz until smooth.

Step 2

Add the almond flour, coconut flour, chia seeds, protein powder, and 1 tbsp of the desiccated coconut and stir together well until the mixture resembles bread crumbs.

Step 3

Add the melted coconut oil, then the honey, and mix well.

Step 4

Roll into 10 small balls using your hands.

Step 5

Spread the remaining desiccated coconut on the kitchen worktop and then roll the balls in it.

Delicious Dates Bites

Ingredients

1 cup of medjool dates, pitted

3/4 cup almonds

3/4 cup walnuts

2 tbsp chia seeds

1 tbsp coconut oil

1 scoop chocolate protein powder

1 tbsp of organic raw cacao powder

Servings - 8

Calories: 246

Protein: 8g

Carbs: 21g

Fat: 17g

Step 1

Add the almonds, walnuts and chia seeds to a food processor and blend until a flour consistency has been created.

Step 2

Add all the remaining ingredients and blend until a sticky dough has formed.

Step 3

Roll the dough intol balls, place in a plastic tub, and store in the fridge.

Protein Raisin Cookies

Ingredients

Servings - 6

3 scoops chocolate protein powder

Nutrition per serving

200ml canned butter beans

1 tbsp unsweetened natural peanut butter

Calories: 168

Handful of raisins

Protein: 16g

2 tbsp oats

Carbs: 16g

2 tbsp Greek yoghurt

Fat: 5g

1 tbsp coconut oil

Step 1

Preheat the oven to 150°C/300°F/gas 2.

Step 2

Add all ingredients in a blender and blitz until blend until a dough is created. If too dry, add a little almond milk or another tbsp of yoghurt.

Step 3

Separate the dough into six balls and flatten with the palms of your hands.

Step 4

Place some parchment paper in a baking tin and add the cookies. Cook in the oven for 10-12 minutes or until golden brown.

Almond Fudge Bars

Ingredients

2 scoops vanilla or chocolate protein powder

1.5 cup oats

2 tbsp almond butter

2 tbsp honey

1 cup Rice Crispies cereal

1 tsp vanilla extract

2 tbsp almond milk

Servings - 6

Nutrition per serving

Calories: 233

Protein: 13g

Carbs: 36g

Fat: 5g

Step 1

Add a sheet of parchment paper to a casserole dish / baking tray.

Step 2

Grind 1 cup of oats into a flour consistency and then add to a large mixing bowl, along with another 1/2 cup of oats, protein powder and Rice Crispies cereal.

Step 3

Put a small saucepan on a low-medium heat and melt the almond butter. Then mix in the honey and vanilla extract, stirring for 2-3 mins.

Step 4

Remove from the heat and add to the other ingredients in the mixing bowl, stirring well until they are combined.

Step 5

Using a wooden spoon, transfer the mixture into the cooking dish / baking tray and flatten in evenly with the palms of your hands.

Step 6

Place in the fridge for 45-60 mins and then cut into separate bars.

Healthy Shakes

- **A blender (not a juicer) is essential. You can find a decent one online via Amazon for around £30.**

- **Simply chuck all ingredients in these recipes in blender and blitz for 1 minute until smooth.**

- **The first three recipes are intentionally higher in calories for people looking to gain weight and muscle mass
(instructions are also provided to reduce the calorie count).**

- **Again, I recommend <u>plant-based</u> protein powders (i.e. Sunwarrior or Vegan Blend from MyProtein.com)
rather than whey protein powder with these recipes.**

Blueberry Blast

Ingredients

Handful of frozen blueberries

1/2 ripe banana

1 scoop of chocolate protein powder

Half tin (200ml) coconut milk

2 tbsp oats

1/4 tsp cinnamon

Cup of water

2 or 3 ice cubes

Nutrition per shake

Calories: 850

Protein: 30g

Carbs: 73g

Fat: 49g

(Using only 1/4 tin of coconut milk instead will reduce the calories by around 150-170).

Choc n' Banana

Ingredients

1 ripe banana

1 scoop choc protein powder

1 tbsp unsweetened peanut butter

Handful of almonds / mixed nuts

1 tbsp oats

1 tbsp linseed

1/4 tsp cinnamon

Cup of water

2 or 3 ice cubes

Nutrition per shake

Calories: 685

Protein: 40g

Carbs: 58g

Fat: 33g

(Using only 1 tbsp of peanut butter will reduce calories by 100-150).

Mango Monster

Ingredients

1 cup of frozen mango

1 scoop of chocolate protein powder

Half can (200ml) coconut milk

2 tbsp linseed

2 tbsp sunflower seeds

1/4 tsp ginger and/or nutmeg

Handful of spinach

Cup of water

2 or 3 ice cubes

Nutrition per shake

Calories: 900

Protein: 39g

Carbs: 33g

Fat: 69g

* (Using only 1/4 tin of coconut milk will reduce the calories by around 150-170).

Avocado Attack

Ingredients

2 tbsp of oats

Half an avocado

Handful of pumpkin seeds

1 tbsp of peanut butter

1 scoop of protein powder

1-1.5 cups of water

Nutrition per shake

Calories: 600

Protein: 37g

Carbs: 42g

Fat: 32g

Strawberry Goji Smooth

Ingredients

1 scoops of strawberry protein powder

2 cups of unsweetened almond milk (or water)

3 fresh strawberries

1-2 tsp goji powder

2 or 3 ice cubes

Nutrition per shake

Calories: 262

Protein: 18g

Carbs: 24g

Fat: 9g

Tropical Twist

Ingredients

1 scoop of vanilla or plain protein powder

1/4 cup frozen pineapple chunks

1/2 frozen banana

1/2 cup frozen mango chunks

1 cup of almond milk (or water)

2 or 3 ice cubes

Nutrition per shake

Calories: 220

Protein: 28g

Carbs: 53g

Fat: 7g

Green Pineapple Power

Ingredients	**Nutrition per shake**
½ cup unsweetened almond milk	Calories: 420
⅓ cup nonfat plain Greek yogurt	Protein: 12g
1 cup baby spinach	Carbs: 55g
1 frozen banana	Fat: 18g
½ cup frozen pineapple chunks	
1 tablespoon chia seeds	
1-2 tsps of honey	

Ginger Booster

Ingredients

200g Greek natural yoghurt

1 frozen banana

2 tbsp almond butter

1 tsp ground ginger

1/4 tsp ground cinnamon

Cup of water

2 or 3 ice cubes

Nutrition per shake

Calories: 528

Protein: 17g

Carbs: 41g

Fat: 35g

Chia Berry

Ingredients

200g Greek natural yoghurt

1 frozen banana

100g blueberries

3 or 4 large strawberries

1/4 tsp ground ginger

Cup of water

2 or 3 ice cubes

Nutrition per shake

Calories: 422

Protein: 11g

Carbs: 54g

Fat: 20g

Tropical Treat

Ingredients

1 scoop vanilla protein powder

300ml pineapple juice

1/2 frozen banana

2 tbsp Greek yoghurt

3 or 4 large strawberries

2 or 3 ice cubes

Nutrition per shake

Calories: 336

Protein: 12g

Carbs: 58g

Fat: 7g

About the author

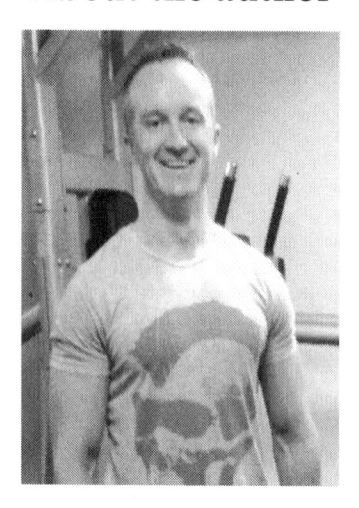

Marc McLean is a 30 something year old online personal training and nutrition coach from Loch Lomond in Scotland. He owns Weight Training Is The Way and is a health and fitness writer for leading websites including The Good Men Project, Mind Body Green, and Healthgreatness.com

Marc loves...climbing Munros (aka the biggest hills) in Scotland, peanut butter, amazing scenery, the Rocky movies, lifting heavy things, blueberries, Daft Punk, watching tennis, travelling and laughing. Not in that particular order.

Marc hates...bad manners, funerals, cardio, and all drivers who don't indicate.

You can connect with Marc here:

Email: marc@weighttrainingistheway.com

Website: www.weighttrainingistheway.com

Facebook: www.facebook.com/weighttrainingistheway

Instagram: www.instagram.com/weight_training_is_the_way